What's Really in Our Bread?

By David Upthegrove

For my parents

What's Really in Our Bread?

Introduction

This book was written to help young readers learn about the food we eat, especially bread and to spark curiosity about where food comes from and how it affects our bodies. Bread is something many of us eat every day, so it makes a great place to start asking questions: How does wheat grow? What happens on farms? What do farmers use to protect crops — and why might that matter to us?

We'll explore one common example, a weed killer called glyphosate, which is also used to speed up crop drying times. This information is not to frighten you, but to show how chemicals used in farming can sometimes end up in soil, water, and food. Scientists are still learning exactly what long-term, small amounts of these chemicals do to our bodies. That's why asking questions, reading carefully, and learning how food is grown are important skills. Knowledge is power: the more we understand the better choices we can make for our health.

The language is simple; the ideas are explained in short chapters. My hope is to inspire curiosity, not fear, to encourage you to explore, experiment, and discover how a clean food supply helps bodies grow strong and minds stay sharp.

This story begins with three curious kids, a golden wheat field, and a question, what's really in our bread?

The goal of this book is not to frighten readers but to encourage curiosity and careful thinking. Mary, Ben, and Ana follow clues and   ask adults thoughtful questions. Along the way they learn how food moves from farm to table and how communities can work together to make change.

If this book raises questions you'd like to explore with children, there is an educator/parent guide with activities, sources, and classroom experiments available.

What's Really in Our Bread?

Table of Contents

Chapter 1 — The Golden Wheat Field

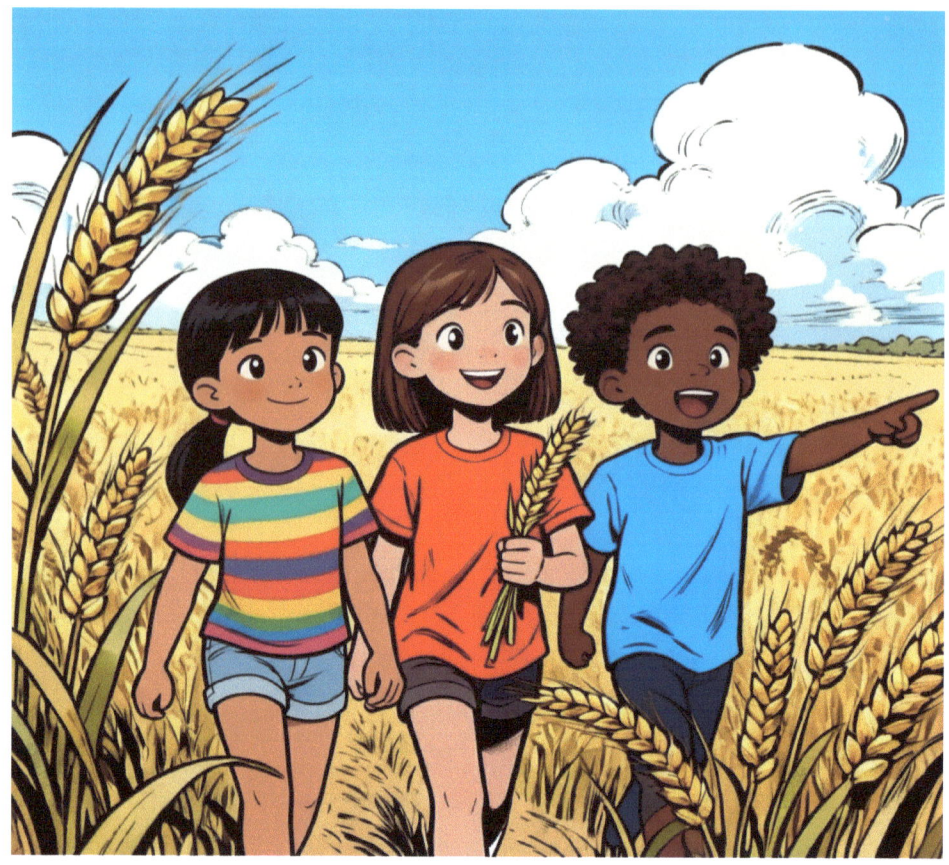

Mary, Ana, and Ben ran through the wheat like it was their own secret kingdom. The tall stalks brushed their shoulders and tickled their legs. Sun warmed the tops of the fields until the whole place looked like a rolling ocean of gold.

Mary loved to learn. She was ten and asked a lot of questions, especially about how things were made. Today she held a wheat stalk in her hand and turned it over, examining the tiny grains as if they were treasures.

"Grandma says this wheat becomes flour, and flour becomes bread!" Mary announced, her brown hair dancing with every step.

Ben, who was nine and always ready for a joke, pretended to be a pirate. "A treasure of bread! Arrr!" He laughed and took a long, dramatic sniff. "It smells like… warm cookies." His grin was wide and trusting.

Ana listened more quietly. She stood still and closed her eyes, breathing in the breeze. "I like how it sounds," she said. "When I run a hand through it, it whispers."

Mary, "Do you think your Grandma will make cinnamon rolls today?"

Ben asked hopefully.

Mary thought of Grandma's kitchen: flour on the table, the other ingredients on the counter top, the way Grandma pinched the dough and laughed.

The memory made her chest warm. "Maybe," she said. "Grandma always says wheat is magic."

They played hide-and-seek among the stalks and dared each other to find the tallest plant. The field felt safe and real—until it didn't.

At the edge of the field a small sign said 'Local Farm Cooperative.' Mary made a note to ask Grandma where the farm sold its grain. That small plan would matter later, they didn't know it yet.

A low rumble interrupts their peaceful day.

Chapter 2 — The Boom Sprayer Arrives

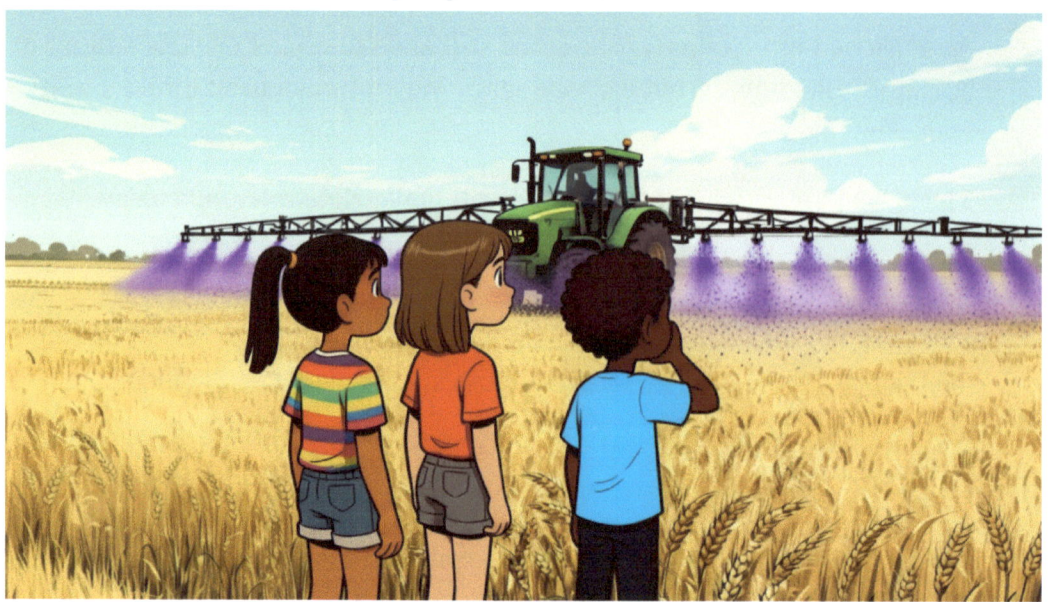

The first sound was a low, mechanical rumble that didn't belong in a field.

The three kids stopped and looked toward the road where dust was rising. A large machine rolled up between the rows—a tractor with long metal arms stretching out like airplane wings.

"It's huge," Ben whispered, stepping closer.

Mary squinted at the letters on the side. "Boom Sprayer," she read aloud. The machine began spraying a fine mist over all the beautiful wheat. The mist settled on every plant, every grain, covering everything in the field.

Ben wrinkled his nose as the mist passed by. It smelled faintly of chemicals, sharp and unfamiliar. "It stings my nose," he said.

Mary, Ana and Ben looked at each other with confused faces. Something didn't feel right.

"Why are they doing that?" Ben asked.

Ana, exclaimed," Let's get out of here!"

But before they could leave, they noticed something strange. There were two men and a woman standing on the road at the edge of the field, talking and smiling. They wore suits and shiny shoes that didn't belong in a farm field.

The children could hear the executives talking.

"Spray it all with glyphosate, (pronounced GLY-fo-sate)",”they heard one of the men say out loud. . The word rolled in the air like something important and secret.

“This will dry the wheat out fast so we can harvest two weeks early.

 “But sir,” said one of the business men, “what about safety concerns?”

The man laughed coldly. “That’s not our problem.

We need to maximize profits. The customers will never know what we used to speed things up. Time is money."”

Mary felt uneasy. The wheat had been a promise—bread, cookies, Grandma’s cinnamon rolls. The thought that something invisible might be on those golden grains made her chest tighten.

The men in suits drove away and the machines finished spraying. The field was left smelling faintly of chemicals.

Chapter 3 — The Wheat Changes

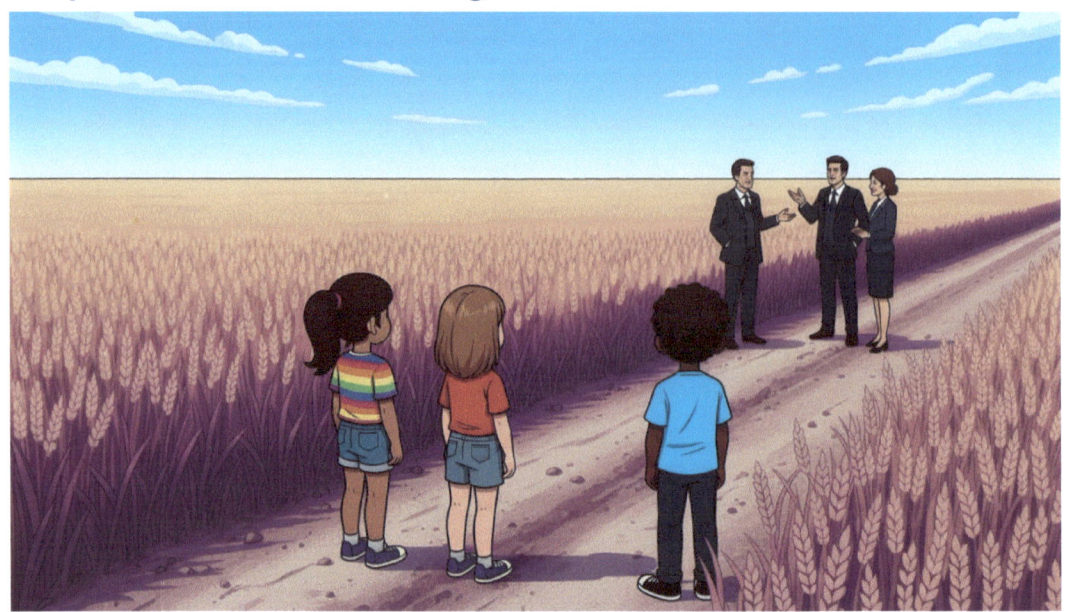

When the children returned a few days later, the field looked different. The waves of gold were patchy and dry. Stalks leaned sideways.

"Mary!" Ben gasped. "The wheat looks… different somehow!" The wheat had dried out much faster than normal and looked withered.

"Mary, it looks… tired," Ben said.

Mary ran a hand along a stalk and imagined it purple in her mind—a color she used to picture things she couldn't see, like a way to make invisible things visible. "It's like the wheat is sick," Ana said quietly, touching a dried stalk.

"Ben, I think ALL wheat gets sprayed like this, not just this field."

"All of it?" Ben asked with wide eyes. "I think so. The chemical they sprayed - glyphosate - it's used everywhere to make wheat dry faster so companies can harvest it quicker.

Near the edge of the field, they saw the same men in suits; they were all looking at papers and calculators. "Excellent!" one of them said, rubbing his hands together greedily. "The glyphosate worked perfectly. We are harvesting two weeks ahead of schedule. That's millions more in profit this quarter!"

"What about the chemical residue on the wheat?", asked the woman with them.

The first man shrugged. "Not our concern. We're in the business of fast harvests and big profits. The processing plants will handle it from here. Besides, it's legal - the government allows it."

"Look," the man said impatiently, "we use these chemicals to speed up production and maximize profits. That's business. If people don't like it, they can buy organic - but that costs more, and most people just want cheap food."

A farmer passing by in a truck stopped to say hello and talk to the children. Ben asked the farmer," Do all of the wheat fields look like this?" "You think all wheat is sprayed?" Ana asked. He sighed. "Lots of commercial wheat farms use desiccants, (pronounced Dess ih kants), now. It makes the harvest easier.

It's what the corporations want." He sounded tired, almost apologetic. "The majority of people don't always know how wheat is grown, harvested or processed, so the companies get away with it."

Mary grabbed Ben's hand. "Come on, let's follow the wheat and see what happens to it."

Chapter 4 — Harvest and the Convoy

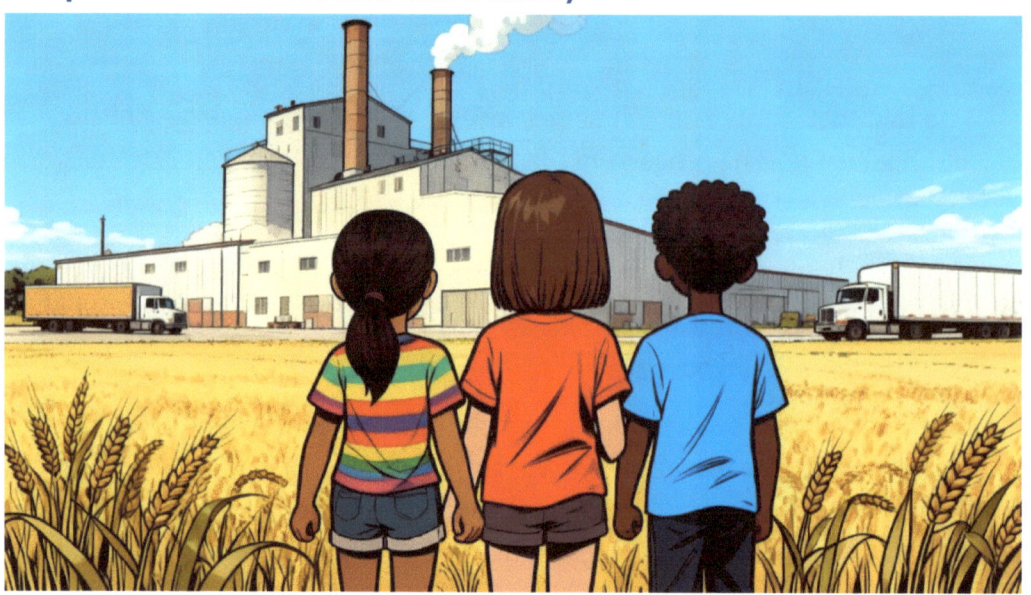

Harvest machines rolled onto the fields to collect the wheat. The machines, called combines were huge. The kids watched from the side of the road as combines mowed down the stalks and spit out straw. Trucks were lined up like a convoy, ready to take loads of freshly harvested wheat to the processing mill.

A truck driver was standing outside of his truck. The children ran up to him to ask about the machines. "You shouldn't be near the road, kids," he said at first, but then his tone softened. "You see all this? It's county-wide harvesting.

Ana asked the truck driver," What are the machines doing?"

"The harvester cuts the wheat stalks and then separates the grain from the chaff. Then the grain is sifted to remove any other debris. The cleaned grain is stored in these tanks. We haul it to the mill, it is turned into flour."

"What about the glyphosate on the wheat," Mary asked.

"It stays on the wheat and almost all of the wheat these days gets the same chemical treatment before it is harvested."

"Doesn't it bother anyone?" Ben asked.

He shrugged. "We're paid to deliver the wheat. People higher up make the decisions about how the wheat is grown, treated and harvested."

The convoy rolled away toward a cluster of buildings with tall chimneys. Mary felt the weight of everything—wheat going from field to mill to grocery—and imagined the people who would someday eat whatever came out of those buildings. Her stomach tightened. "We have to see inside of the mill," she said.

Later that afternoon, they made a plan to visit the mill. The three friends rode their bikes up to the flour mill. Mary, Ana and Ben stood outside of the mills' side entrance looking for an opportunity to look inside.

Chapter 5 — The Flour Mill

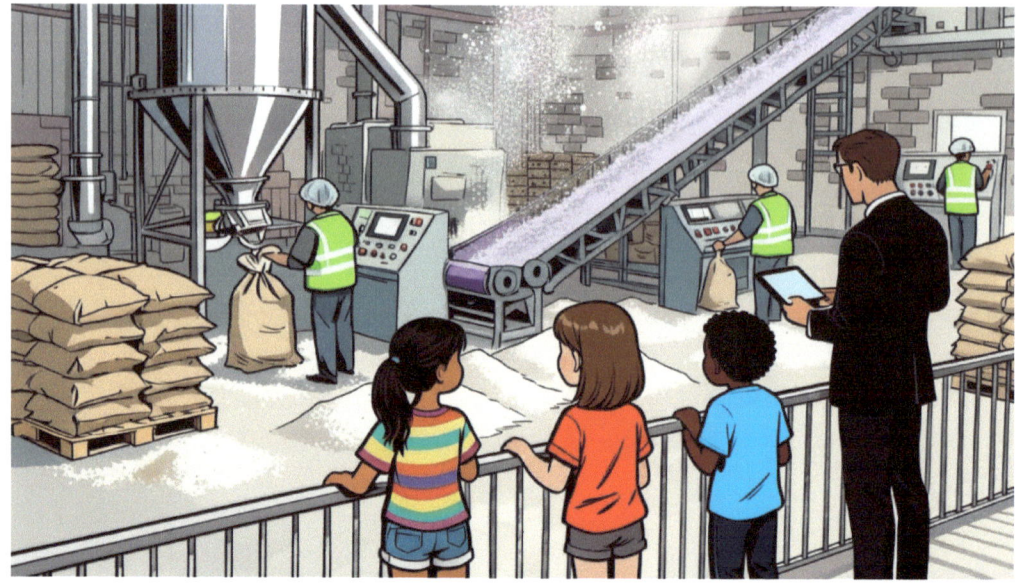

The side entrance door opened and a couple of workers walked out past the three children. Another worker was standing by the door waiting to go inside. Ben got his attention, he asked," Mister, can we see what happens to the wheat?" The man responded, "You can come inside with me, there is an observation platform located inside the mill just past the doorway." Mary, Ana and Ben looked into a room full of conveyor belts, roller mills, grain cleaners, sifters, blending machines. . The grains from the wheat poured into machines, and then a fine pale powder came out of the sifters.

"Wow," Ana exclaimed. Mary and Ben stood in awe. The noise vibrated their bodies.

"The contamination is in all the flour!" Ben exclaimed.

Ben noticed that is was not pure while but slightly brown. Mary imagined it looked kind of purple.

Flour dust hung in the air, and the big machines packaging the flour made the room seem even bigger.

The workers moved with quick efficiency. A supervisor checked his watch and pointed. A conveyor rolled sacks toward a machine that filled them with flour a robotic arm separated the bags for stacking.

"Why is the flour so white?" Ben asked the foreman.

A man in a blue coat, his palms dusted, looked at the children and hesitated. He looked like someone who had seen many nights and early mornings. "Sir!" Ben asked, "What happens to the wheat here?"

The worker stopped and turned. He wiped his hands on his coat. "Kids," he said, "this place turns wheat into flour."

We clean it, grind it, and sometimes we treat it so it looks consistent. Bleaching agents, conditioners—things to make it bake the same every time. They say it's to meet standards."

Ana, Mary and Ben watched in horror as chemicals were added to make the flour look white, the contamination was still there just hidden and invisible.

"What about the glyphosate residue from the drying process?" Mary asked, thinking about the mist from the sprayer.

He looked away as if the question had a taste he didn't like. "Yes," it does and I worry, about how that might affect my family and other people.

The chemical companies say it's safe, the government allows it, and we just do our jobs. Treat it and bleach it white then ship it out." Profits are what it's all about.

I do what I have to do to keep my job. But I can tell you this; if you really want to change things, tell more people that care about how their food is grown and processed

As they walked back to the exit from the observation area, a security guard was standing next to the door with a clipboard and a stern face said, "This area is off-limits," he said. "You kids can't be wandering around here." The guard's voice was firm, but not unkind.

Mary felt relief that they were able to see the way wheat was processed and talk to one of the employees. The children's questions were answered.

"We're learning," she said. "We just want to know what happens to the wheat after it is harvested."

He sighed and offered a small concession. "There's a public notice board at the mill entrance. It lists where the grain comes from and what kinds of safety reports are filed. You can look there, but stay out of the restricted areas."

Ben squinted at the guard and then at the mill. The restricted area was an obstacle, but they were able to get the needed information. Now they would go to the public notice board to gather more facts.

Chapter 6 — Bread Making and Fast Food

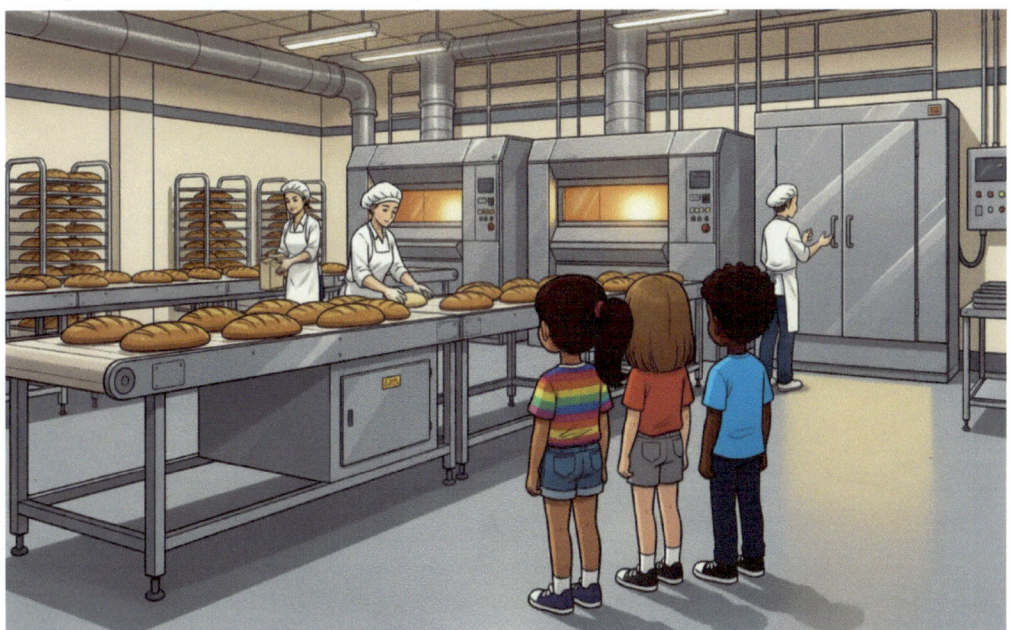

The flour from the mill was used in all kinds of kitchens.

At Amazing Bread Bakery the ovens glowed and the bakers shaped loaves with practiced hands. The bread smelled familiar and warm, the way Mary remembered from Grandma's house, but now she thought of the glyphosate used in the growing process and how it remains in the flour after the wheat is processed into flour.

A truck from the mill backed up to loading dock, and workers unloaded bags of flour. "Faster, faster!" a foreman called to the workers. "We've got orders."

Inside of the bakery, bags of flour were poured into machines where flour was mixed into dough. That dough was used in the baking machines that produced loaves of bread sold in grocery stores. In another part of the bakery hamburger buns, hot dog buns, and sandwich rolls were made from the same flour.

Mary and Ana watched from a safe distance as bread rolled down an assembly line. Each loaf of bread was perfectly shaped. It traveled down a conveyor where the loaf was bagged and placed in shipping trays. Each tray was stacked and ready to ship to grocery stores.

"It looks so normal," Ben whispered.

"But we know what's really in it," Mary said sadly. "And this is happening at every bakery, and the flour is used in every food factory."

Mary watched a baker slide a tray of specialty breads into the oven. He paused when he noticed her interest and smiled kindly. "We try to keep tradition alive," he said. "But these days, we have to use commercially available flour." "My family baked for generations using organic ingredients," he said. "But cheap, fast and big profits are the corporate way."

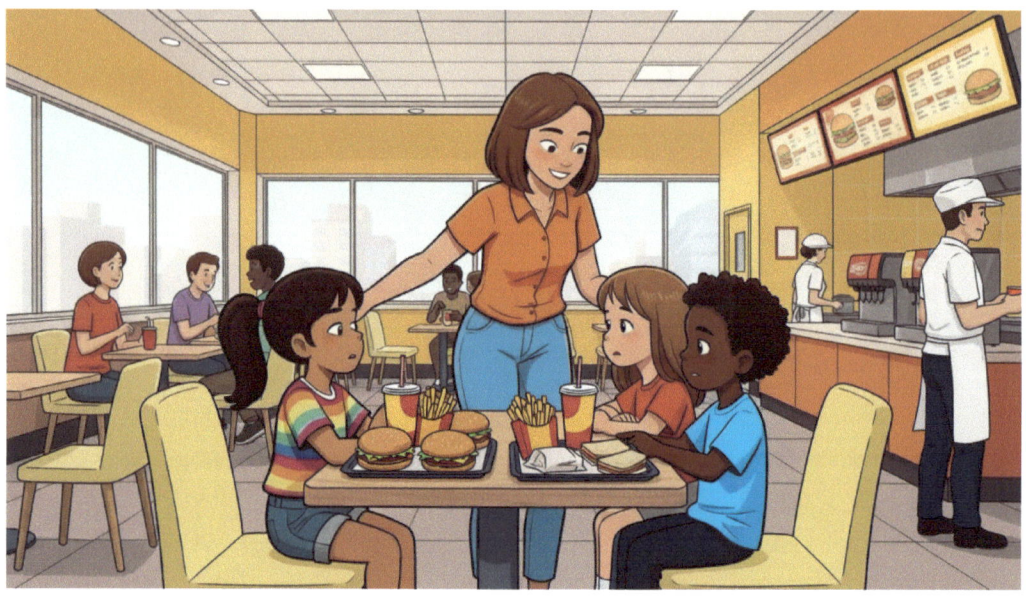

Later that day Mary's mom took Mary, Ana and Ben to a fast food restaurant. Ana noticed a delivery truck from the bakery at the back of the building. Ana said to Ben," even the chicken nuggets are coated in contaminated flour.

Inside the restaurant Ben overheard the manager who was watching the line and tapping his foot.

"Make it fast. Make it cheap," he told his staff. "That's how we stay open."

Kids in the restaurant laughed and traded fries. The smell of warm bread and frying oil made the place feel like any other regular afternoon. Mary thought of all of the families having lunch, stopping in at places that were quick and inexpensive. She understood why people chose these options; sometimes there simply wasn't time to cook from scratch.

Mary realized the problem wasn't just one commercial factory or a secret plan to hurt people. It was a system of choices—some made by people who needed money and some made by companies focused on scale.

Chapter 7 — The Grocery Store

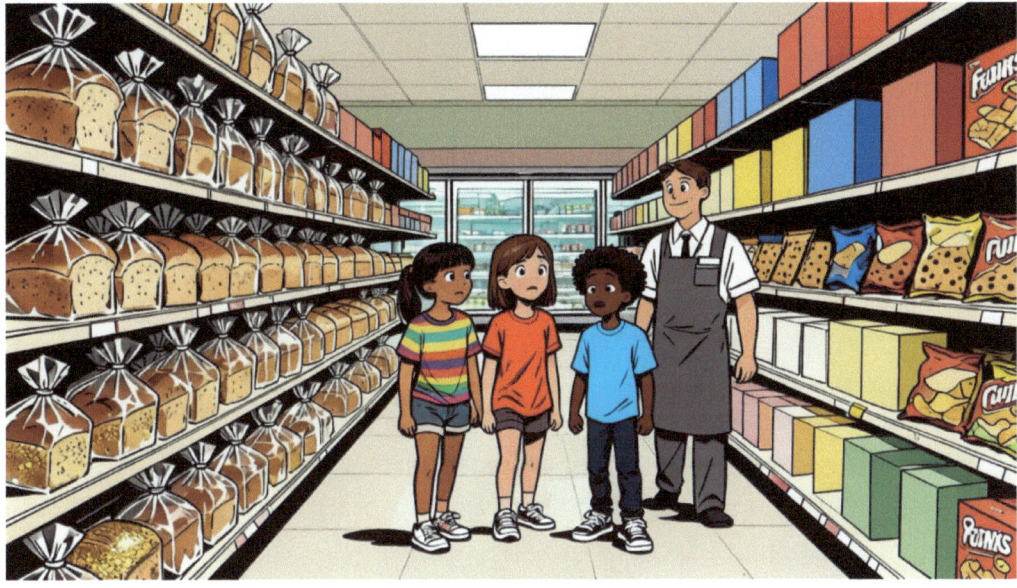

The grocery store shelves were a map of names and logos. Mary ran her fingers down boxes of cereal and rows of bread. "Look at all these brands!" Mary said, reading the labels. "Every popular brand on these shelves all use regular commercial flour." "And cookies!" Ben added. Don't forget cereal,"

Mary continued. "All of the cereals in these colorful boxes with cartoon characters are made with the contaminated flour.

Ana said," Don't forget the pasta and all of those tasty snacks!"

"Even the frozen foods," Mary noticed. "Pizza, chicken nuggets, fish sticks…"Which of these are from the mill?" she wondered aloud.

Ben pointed to a loaf. "Everything that doesn't say organic probably came from regular flour," he said, remembering the worker's warning.

A store clerk noticed their interest and stopped to help. He lowered his voice when they asked where the wheat came from. "Labels help," he told them. "If it says organic, it's grown without synthetic pesticides and certain chemical treatments. People buy what fits their budgets."." But organic costs more

The big companies want everything fast and cheap. Mary's heart sank a little. Bread was a day-to-day thing for many families. If most affordable options came from the same system, then not everyone could choose the organic option.

They filled a small basket with different brands and labels to compare at home. It felt like detective work—reading words, spotting differences, noting what things promised.

At the checkout, Mary tried to memorize a supplier code on the label. It was a jumble of letters and numbers that meant little to her, but it might help if she could match it to the mill list.

Leaving the store, Mary noticed a woman on the sidewalk talking to her child saying, "We can't afford organic every week. Mary sighed, feeling the weight of choices communities face.

Chapter 8 — The School Cafeteria

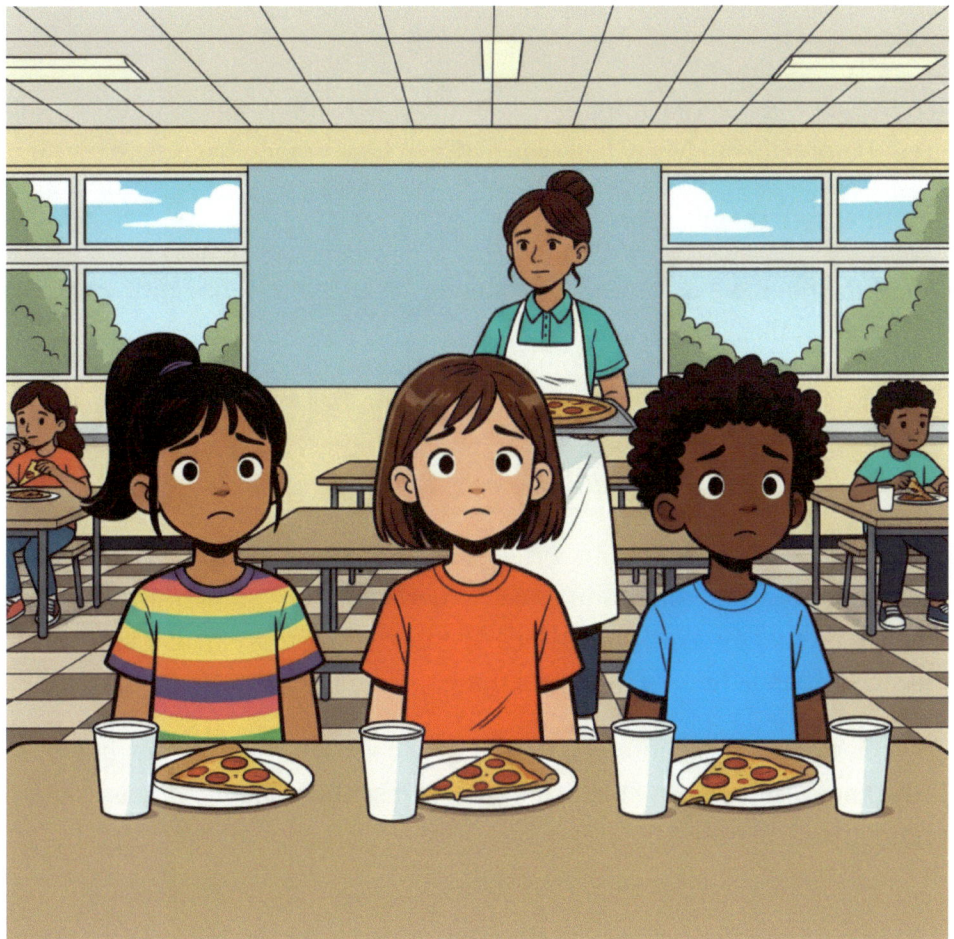

Pizza day arrived with the same cheering as always. The cafeteria warmed with children's chatter and the clatter of trays. Mary, Ana and Ben watched their friends with a new kind of attention, like scientists taking notes. Mary and Ben watched their friends eating happily:

Emma, who had blonde hair and freckles, bit into her peanut butter and jelly sandwich on regular bread,. Jamal, a boy with dark skin and a bright smile ate chicken nuggets Sofia, who spoke Spanish at home, enjoyed her spaghetti made with regular pasta. Kevin, who wore glasses, ate crackers with his soup.

 "They all look so happy," Ana said sadly.

They don't know that almost all this food is made from wheat that was sprayed with chemicals to make companies more money," Mary replied, feeling worried about their friends.

Even the teachers were eating the same food. Mr. Johnson had a turkey sandwich on regular bread, and Ms. Chen was eating a bagel made from conventional flour.

"Should we tell them?" Ben asked.

"Would they believe us?" Mary wondered. "And even if they did, where would they buy food that's different?"

When Mary tried to tell Emma about the wheat, her friend rolled her eyes. "That's gross. I like pizza day." Others shrugged. "Not everything can be organic," a boy named Kevin said. "It's expensive."

The kids learned something important that day: knowing didn't mean others would act on it. Sometimes adults were tired and busy; sometimes the choices depended on money. And sometimes people needed more than a story from a few children to change how things were done.

But when two friends confessed that they had more stomachaches lately, Mary felt the knot inside her tighten. This wasn't just about labels. It was about people feeling unwell and not knowing why.

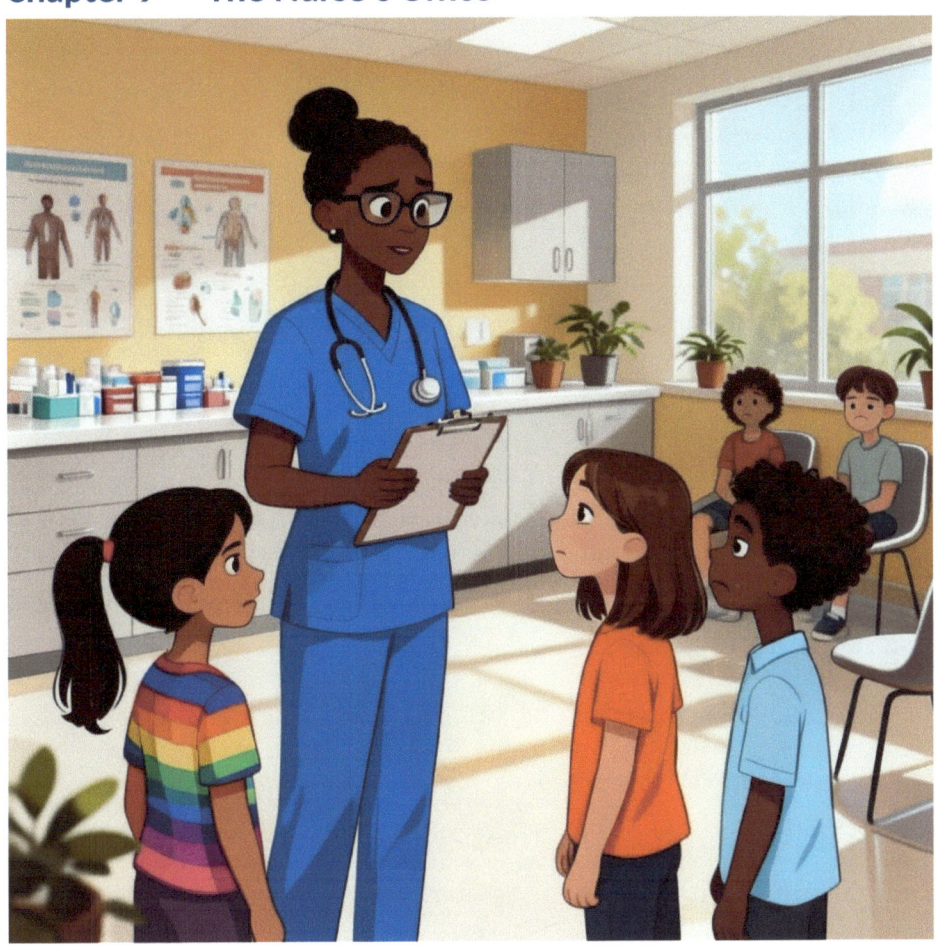

After lunch Mary, Ana and Ben walked by the School nurse's office on their way to class.

Mrs. Patterson's office was bright and cheerful. The nurse looked kind and a little tired. Mary had seen her give ice packs and put bandages on hurt knees for years, but recently the office had been busier with complaints about stomachaches and headaches. Mary said hello to Mrs. Patterson and asked how she was doing.

"This week has been the worst," Mrs. Patterson admitted, pushing her glasses up her nose. "A lot of students have said their tummies hurt after lunch."

"Do you think it could be something in the food?" Mary asked. ."

Mrs. Patterson hesitated and then nodded. "I don't know for sure, but the patterns seem to indicate that it might. It started to look too consistent to be only viruses. I've been keeping notes and telling the school staff."

Ana told Mrs. Patterson that she, Mary and Ben had been investigating the connection between food and people getting sick. Ben passed her a list they had made of symptoms and when they happened. She read it and then smiled sadly. "Kids, you're doing the right thing by taking notes.

Mrs. Patterson showed them a binder she kept with notes about the cafeteria menu and complaints from children. She asked if they would help collect names and dates of any children with health issues. She also advised the students on simple steps to keep their tummies comfortable, like drinking water and choosing fruits and vegetables when possible.

"Why not change the cafeteria food," Ben asked.

Mrs. Patterson replied," Changing a school's menu is complicated and expensive. Sometimes the district chooses what they can afford."

The nurse promised to speak to the cafeteria manager and the principal if more students and their families reported continuing symptoms. That promise was small but it was a chance to do something about the children's discoveries about bread and other food contaminated with chemicals. Now there was a chance that the children could work with the adults who could act.

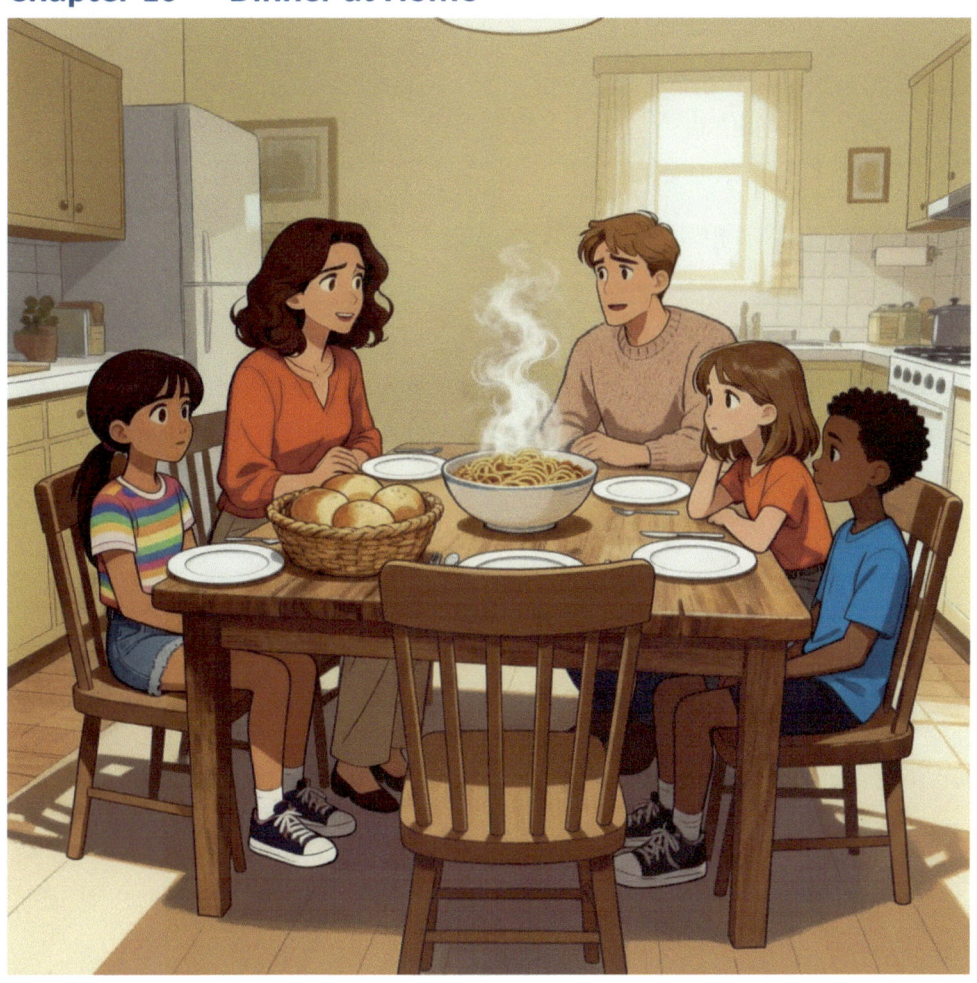

Dinner that night was spaghetti with garlic bread. Grandma's recipe was always a family favorite. The smell made Mary's mouth water, but then she remembered contaminated flour. She noticed Ana and Ben look slightly concerned.

"Why aren't you eating much, kids?" Mary's dad asked, noticing their hesitation.

"Mom, Dad," Mary said," We learned something important. Do you know that almost all wheat is sprayed with a chemical called glyphosate to make it dry faster so companies can harvest it quicker and make more money?" "We learned that a lot of wheat gets sprayed before it's harvested and might leave something on the wheat."

 "What?" Mom looked surprised. "I had no idea."

"It's true," Ben added. "The chemical stays on the wheat even after it becomes flour and bread."

Her parents exchanged a look. "How do you know?" Dad asked, curious but careful.

"We saw the sprayer," Ben said. "We saw trucks going to the mill. A farmer told us that all commercial wheat growers spray the wheat to make it dry faster. A worker from the mill told us they treat the flour to make it look white. We talked to the nurse at school, too."

Mom folded her hands. "We'll look into it," she said. "Let's try something for a week: we'll buy organic bread and pasta and see if anyone feels different."

For the next few days, the family ate organic bread bought from a small store. Mom kept a list of how everyone felt. Slowly, Dad noticed his headaches seemed less frequent. Mom said she had more energy in the mornings. It wasn't proof of anything, but it was a beginning It was an experiment they could understand.

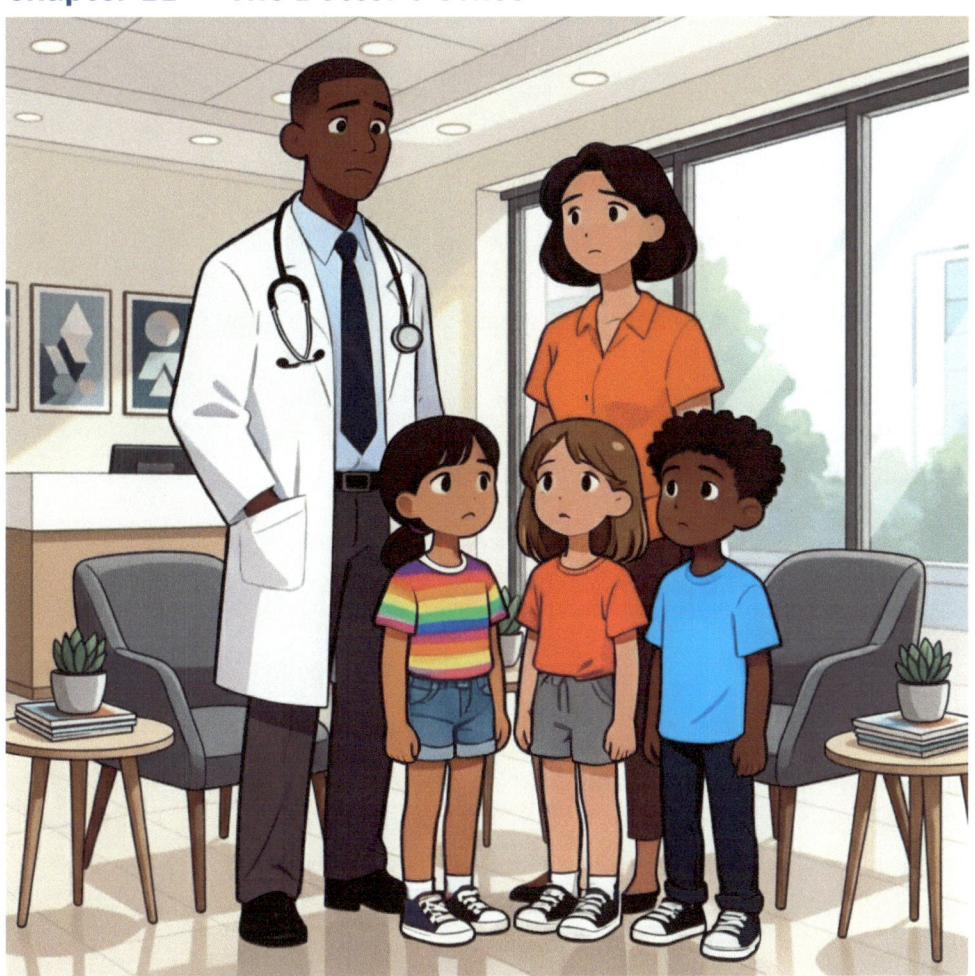

The following Saturday, Mary and Ben found themselves in Dr. Williams'
waiting room with their mom, who wanted to ask about the connection between
food and her symptoms.

The waiting room hummed with soft conversation. The waiting room had several
families waiting, parents holding their stomachs, children looking tired, and
everyone seeming uncomfortable.

"This is concerning," the receptionist said to her colleague. "We're seeing so
many patients with digestive issues and headaches lately."

Mary looked around and recognized some faces from their community,

Dr. Williams came out looking thoughtful. "I'm sorry for the wait everyone.
We're seeing an increase in digestive issues, headaches, and fatigue. I've been
researching possible causes."

When it was their turn, Mom asked, "Doctor, could chemicals used in food production be causing health problems?"

Dr. Williams nodded seriously. "That's actually something I've been investigating. There's growing concern about glyphosate residues in our food supply. Research shows that glyphosate can harm the good bacteria in our stomachs."

The doctor was calm and used simple words for the kids. He explained that inside their tummies lived millions of tiny helpers called good bacteria. Those helpers helped digest food and kept bodies balanced.

Dr. Williams said," Glyphosate the chemical they spray on wheat can kill off up to 40% of these good bacteria," the doctor explained. "When you don't have enough good bacteria, your tummy can't work properly, and you might get stomachaches, headaches, or feel tired."

 Mary's eyes widened. "So the flour made from the chemical sprayed wheat actually hurts the helpful bacteria inside our bodies? "Exactly, Mary, Your gut needs those good bacteria to stay healthy .When chemicals kill them off, it's like losing almost half of your body's cleanup crew."

"Some scientists are studying how certain chemicals might affect those bacteria," Dr. Williams said. "There's ongoing research, and doctors pay attention when patterns of illness in communities change. It's right to ask questions and gather data. Sometimes removing a suspected cause for a while, like trying organic food for a week can helps see if there's a difference."

Ana asked, "Can the bacteria come back?"

"Yes," Dr. Williams answered. "With time and the right foods, like fruits and vegetables your body can rebuild healthy bacteria. If someone feels sick a lot, they should see a doctor. And families can consider food choices and talk to their schools and local stores about options."

Dr. Williams' tone made Mary and Ana feel both cautious and encouraged. There were no simple answers, but the path forward had steps they could take.

Dr. Williams suggests the family keep a simple food-and-symptom diary.

Chapter 12 — The Health Food Store

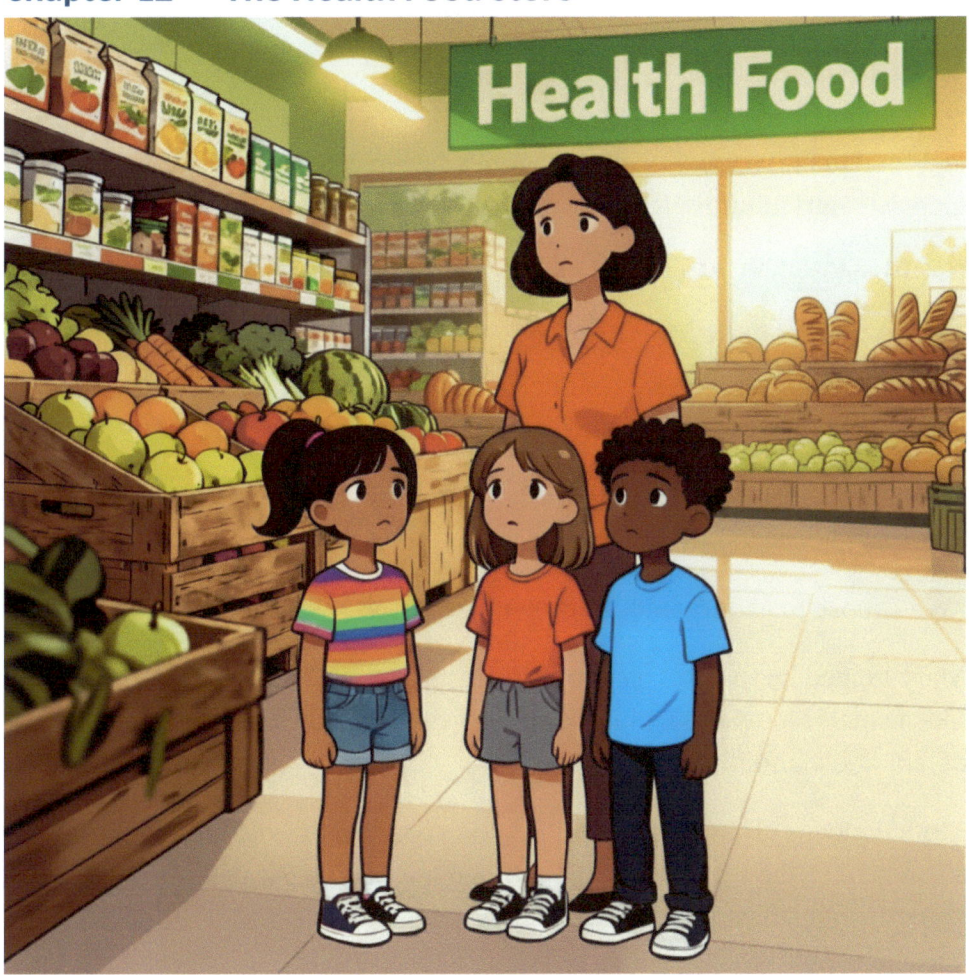

After their doctor visit, Ana, Mary and Ben went with Mary's mom to the health food store to buy organic bread. At the health food store, the organic bread sat in baskets. A radio played quietly.

Mary and her mom were comparing labels when Mary heard two customers talking near the cereal shelf. One said, "My husband is a sales representative for a major chemical company. He said they moved a lot of volume this quarter. Sales were up from farms using their products," Apparently the quarterly profits from their glyphosate division are incredible," the woman said. "Every farm that uses those chemicals to speed up harvesting means more money for the company and a bigger bonus for him."

"What about the health concerns?" the other asked.

"Look, they are not breaking any laws. The government allows it, farmers use it and food manufactures want the harvest faster. They provide a legal product that increases agricultural efficiency and most importantly profits.

Her friend replied, "But most people don't even know about the chemicals."

"That's not my husband's responsibility; they are in business to make money, not educate consumers. Those chemicals are not required to be listed on ingredient labels. As long as it's legal and profitable, they keep selling."

"The market demands cheap, consistent supply. If consumers want chemical-free, they can choose to buy organic."

"We choose to eat organic food as much as possible."

Mary tugged her mom's sleeve and whispered, "did you hear that?". It sounded like a small secret and a big reason why there is a lack of knowledge. Most people do not know about the chemicals.

Mom nodded. "That's why families and communities asking questions can bring awareness to the issue," she said. "If enough people want a different kind of food system, companies will have to change."

It wasn't a villain story where someone had to be punished. It was a complicated system where many people made choices—sometimes because of money, sometimes because of comfort, and sometimes because they didn't know.

Mary felt clearer. Change would take time, and it would need facts, kind open conversations, and people working together.

Chapter 13 — The School Meeting

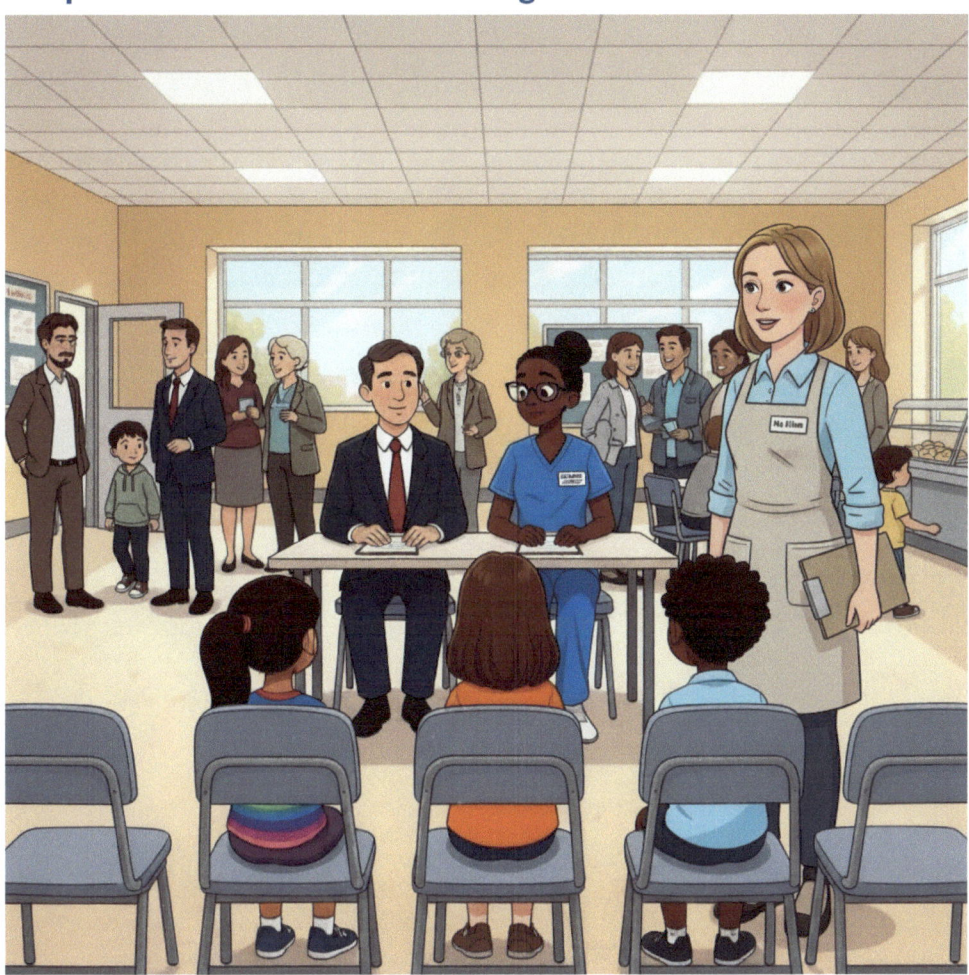

The cafeteria looked different without trays and noise. Folding chairs faced a small table where Mrs. Patterson sat beside the principal, Mr. Alvarez, and the cafeteria manager, Ms. Kline. On a poster board, Mary had pasted simple charts: days of the week on one side; tally marks for tummy aches on the other.

Parents trickled in, some with babies, some holding hands with kids. Mary's stomach fluttered. She wasn't a teacher or a doctor—just a kid who had seen things and written them down.

Mrs. Patterson opened gently. 'We've seen more visits for stomachaches and headaches after lunch this term. We're not jumping to conclusions, but we are listening. Mary and her friends noticed patterns and kept notes. They asked for tonight's meeting to share and to ask for help.'

Mary explained their diary. She didn't say 'danger' or 'blame.' She said, 'We noticed that when we ate certain foods, some of us felt better.' She showed her small chart and passed copies of a one-page flyer that said: 'Try It for a Week: Our School's Gentle Food Experiment.'

Mr. Alvarez cleared his throat. 'Our budget is tight. We buy what we can afford and what the program allows. But if families want to try bringing lunches from home for one week, and if our cafeteria can add one organic option for that week, we can track what happens.'

Ms. Kline nodded. 'We can do one organic whole-wheat bread option for sandwiches next week and label it clearly. We'll take notes too.'

A father raised his hand. 'And if kids feel better, what then?'

'Then we'll look for grants and community partners,' Mrs. Patterson said. "small steps. We start with data we can collect together.'

When the meeting ended, Mary felt lighter. No one promised miracles. But everyone had agreed to try.

A storm cloud rumbles outside; Mary wonders if anyone will actually participate.

Chapter 14 — Pilot Week

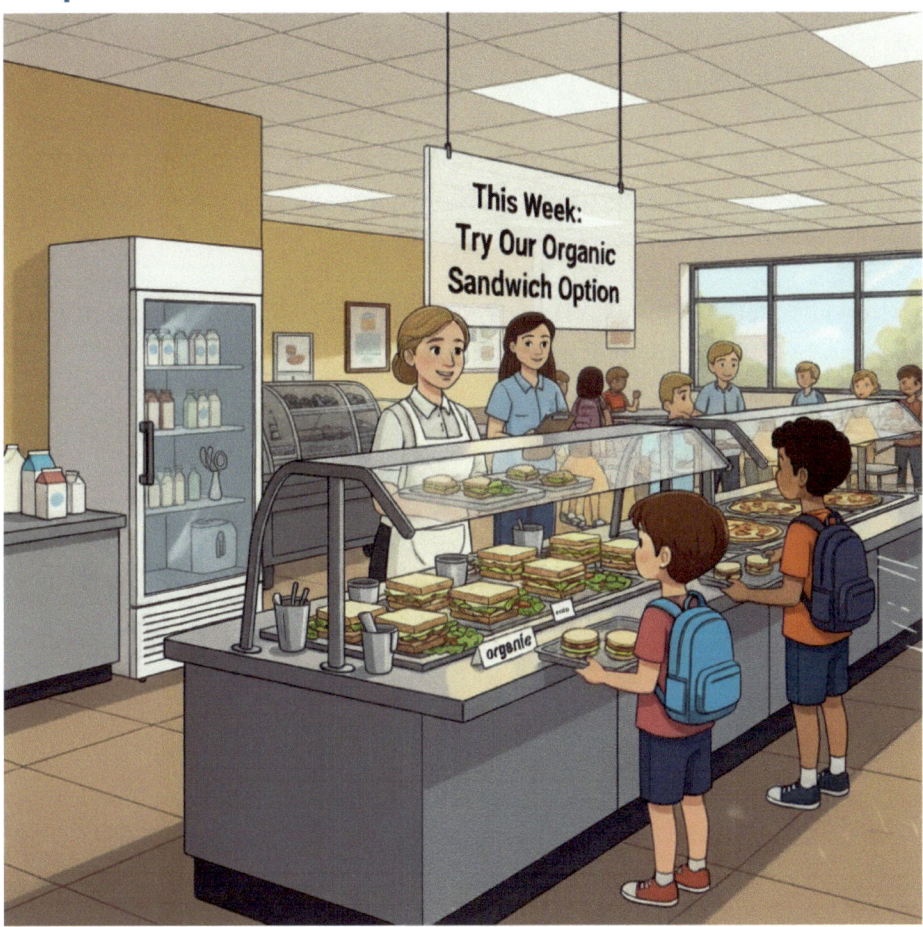

Monday began with a sign above the lunch line: 'This Week: Try Our Organic Sandwich Option.' Ms. Kline wore a nervous smile. The bread looked the same, but the label was new.

Some kids hurried past, pizza on their minds. Others paused. Emma took a sandwich and shrugged. 'It can't hurt to try.' Kevin wrinkled his nose, then grabbed one too after his mom texted, 'Give it a shot.'

Mrs. Patterson stood near the milk cooler with a clipboard. She wasn't spying; she was counting. How many kids chose the option? How many visited her office later?

By Wednesday, the tally marks began to look different. There fewer visits for tummy aches. Not zero, but fewer. The change was small but visible. There was excitement that change was possible. On Friday, Mr. Alvarez met Mary, Ana and Ben in the nurse's office. It appears that the change in diet made a difference.

Ms. Kline's notes showed that the number of students choosing the organic option compared to the decrease in symptoms was significant. Mr. Alvarez said, "We can budget for offering this option once a week starting next month, for starters."

Ms. Kline checked her notes, "if we get a small donation or a grant, the new menu options can be offered the entire school year.'

Mary and her friends grinned. Data had become decisions. Not perfect, but progress.

That afternoon, Mary taped the Pilot Week chart above her desk at home. The lines were messy but honest. She wrote at the top: 'When we ask and act together, small things change.'

Epilogue — What Mary, Ben, and Ana Learned

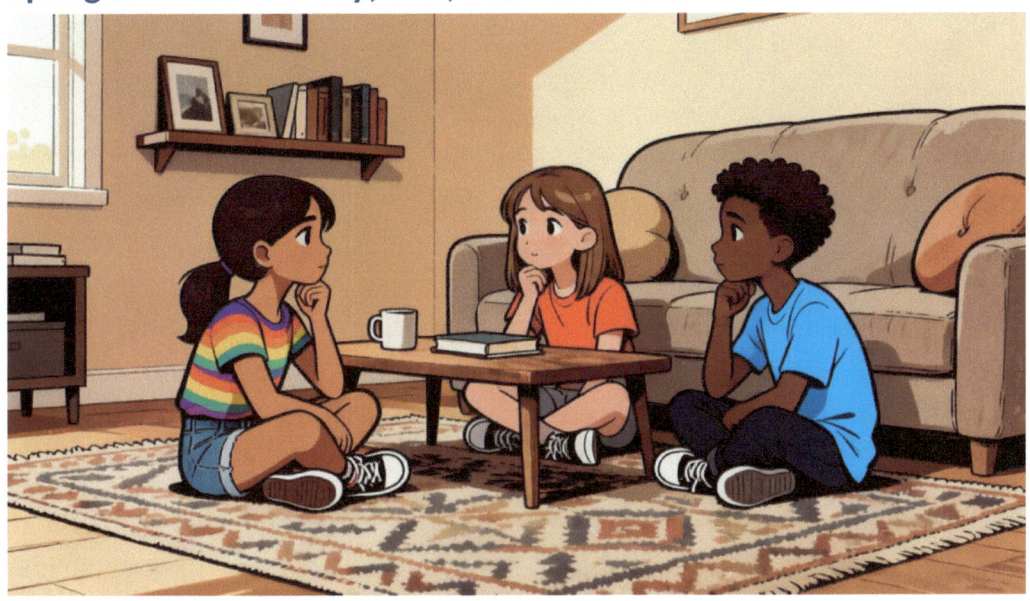

Back in Mary's living room, the three friends sat talking and thinking about everything they had discovered.

"So here's what we know," Mary said, counting on her fingers. "Most commercial wheat farms spray almost all wheat with glyphosate to make it dry faster so they can harvest it quicker and make more money. Those chemicals can stay on the wheat during processing. Flour made from that wheat goes into many foods—bread, pasta, cookies, pizza—and sometimes people get stomach pains, headaches, or feel tired. Doctors are studying this, and some scientists say there might be a link."

And the companies know this but don't care because they're making lots of money

"And most people don't even know it's happening," Ben added sadly.

Ben looked determined. "We're kids, but we can do things. We can tell our families, read labels, and keep notes when someone feels unwell.

 Ben thought for a moment. "Maybe we can tell other kids and their families. And they can choose to buy organic food when they can."

 "You're right!" Ana said, getting excited. "If enough people know the truth and choose healthier options, maybe companies will have to change."

We can ask the school to include more organic options when possible."

"What else can we do", Ana asked.

"We can start by asking questions," Ben suggested.

"Like, 'What's really in our bread?' and 'How was this wheat grown?'

Mary nodded. "Most importantly," Ben said wisely for a nine year old, "we learned that companies sometimes care more about making money fast than keeping people healthy."

"And that just because something is legal doesn't mean it's the best choice for our bodies," Ana added. The children decided that even though they were young, they had an important job: to ask questions, learn about their food, and help their family make healthier choices when possible.

Ana smiled. "We can make posters, talk at the PTA, and ask the grocery store manager about affordable options. We can try to show people what we saw and what we learned."

They made a simple plan: take notes from classmates, talk to families, and continue organic options for school lunches.

Mary looked at her friends and felt a warm, quiet hope. "Change doesn't happen overnight," she said, "but it can start with questions and with people caring enough to act."

"Tomorrow," Mary declared, "we start telling everyone: 'Do you know what's really in our bread and how it's made?" And with that important mission in mind, Ana, Mary and Ben started dreaming of a world where companies would care as much about people's health as they do about profits.

Grandma called to say the cinnamon rolls are ready if they are interested.

THE END

Discussion Questions for Young Readers

Why did the children want to learn more about how wheat is grown?

What steps did Mary, Ben, and Ana take to learn the truth? Were they helpful?

Why did the nurse ask for family notes, and how did that help?

What small actions can families take to learn more about their food?

How can kids' share what they learn without scaring people—how can they be persuasive and kind?

If your school tried a pilot week, what would you measure, and how would you decide what to do next?

Author's Note for Parents & Teachers

This story introduces children to the reality of glyphosate (pronounced - GLY-fo-sate) used in commercial wheat production in an age-appropriate way. It explains how this chemical is used as a desiccant to speed harvesting for increased profits, and how this practice affects the food supply.

The story encourages critical thinking about:

• The widespread use of glyphosate in conventional wheat farming

• How corporate profit motives can conflict with health considerations

• The difference between conventional and organic food production

• Reading food labels and making informed choices

• The importance of asking questions about food sources

• How consumer choices can influence corporate practices

The "purple wheat" serves as a visual metaphor that helps children understand invisible chemical contamination in processed foods.

The story emphasizes that this is a systemic issue affecting most conventional wheat products, not just isolated incidents. This story is intended to introduce children to food systems and to encourage curiosity, critical thinking, and healthy conversations in families and classrooms. The narrative focuses on what children can discover and the practical steps they can take to explore questions about their food.

The book presents concerns about residues on conventional wheat through the perspective of children, community conversations, and medical professionals. It does not attempt to provide exhaustive scientific conclusions. For a detailed discussion of the research, balanced sources, and classroom activities, please see the separate educator and parent guide available as companion for this book.

Glossary

Glyphosate: (pronounced GLY-fo-sate.) An herbicide (weed-killer) used on many farms.

Desiccant: A chemical used to dry crops more quickly before harvest.

Residue: Tiny amounts of a chemical left on food after it is used on a farm.

Organic: Food grown without certain synthetic pesticides or desiccants; organic products have specific certifications.

Mill: A place where grain is ground into flour.

Flour: The powder made from grinding grain; used to make bread, pasta, and many other foods.

Co-formulants: Other ingredients in commercial pesticide products (like surfactants) that help the chemical spread; sometimes they change how the product affects living things.

Bleaching agents: Additives used in flour processing to make flour look whiter and more consistent.

Gut microbiome: The tiny helpers (bacteria and other microbes) that live in our intestines and help digest food and protect health.

Educational Notes

The story introduces the concept of desiccation (using chemicals to dry crops faster) and how food moves from farm to plate.

It emphasizes evidence-gathering: observation, talking with workers/experts, keeping records and small experiments (e.g., trying dietary changes).

The children's approach models civic skills:, asking adults thoughtful questions, collecting information, and proposing practical actions to their school and community.

Teachers can use the story to explore topics: basic food supply chains, reading labels, healthy eating, and how to evaluate sources of information.

Why: Small experiments help us learn what helps our students feel their best.

Thank you for being part of our caring school community!

www.ingramcontent.com/pod-product-compliance
Lightning Source LLC
Chambersburg PA
CBHW041556120626
46551CB00002B/230

9 798993 490403